Battling Breast Cancer as a Man:

The Ultimate Survival Guide

By

Carl B. Wilson

Battling Breast Cancer As A Man

TABLE OF CONTENTS

Chapter 1

Introduction

The reader will learn about breast cancer in men in Chapter 1 of "Battling Breast Cancer as a Man: The Ultimate Survival Guide." The chapter will outline the likelihood that males will get breast cancer and the significance of early detection. The author will also cover the book's objectives, including giving men the knowledge and tools they need to successfully traverse the challenging world of breast cancer treatment and recovery. By the end of the chapter, readers will have a fundamental grasp of the difficulties men with breast cancer face and the insightful information and direction the book will offer.

Outline of male breast cancer

Less than 1% of all breast cancer cases in males are breast cancer, making it a rare condition. The risk factors,

symptoms, and screening choices for breast cancer should all be known to males. Breast cancer in men can manifest itself in the milk ducts or glands of the breast tissue, just like it occurs in women. Men are more likely to develop breast cancer if they have a family history, certain genetic abnormalities, radiation exposure, or liver illness. A lump or enlargement in the breast, changes in the nipple, and skin changes around the breast can all be signs of breast cancer in males. Men's breast cancer is uncommon; thus, it frequently advances to a later stage before being discovered. For males who are at risk, early detection and routine screening are particularly crucial.

Early detection is essential.

For successful therapy and better outcomes, males with breast cancer must be found early. Men should take an active role in their breast health and be aware of the symptoms and signs of the disease because male breast cancer is uncommon and frequently not discovered until it has spread. By performing routine self-exams, men can notice any changes in their breast tissue early on. Men with a higher risk of developing breast cancer, such as those with a family history or genetic mutation, should discuss screening procedures like mammography, ultrasound, or MRI with their doctor. There are more therapy choices, and better odds of successful treatment and survival the earlier breast cancer in men is discovered.

The book's objectives

"Battle Breast Cancer as a Man: The Ultimate Survival Handbook" aims to give men the knowledge, direction, and tools they require to successfully negotiate the challenging world of breast cancer treatment and recovery. The book seeks to give men the confidence to make knowledgeable decisions about their treatment and to take an active role in their breast health. One or more of the book's objectives is:

We present a thorough analysis of the risk factors, symptoms, and screening choices for breast cancer in men.

Describing the various breast cancer treatments that are available, along with any possible adverse effects.

Providing helpful suggestions and methods for coping with the emotional and psychological effects of breast cancer as well as the side effects of treatment.

Addressing the particular difficulties men with breast cancer confront, such as stigma and upholding their manhood.

Supplying help and information for loved ones of males battling breast cancer.

Highlight the most recent developments in the study and treatment of breast cancer and how they might affect males with the disease.

Enabling men to actively participate in their treatment for breast cancer and to speak out for their wants and preferences.

The book's ultimate objective is to support men with breast cancer to achieve the best outcomes and thrive after treatment.

Chapter 2

Knowledge of Breast Cancer

In "Batting Breast Cancer as a Man: The Complete Survival Handbook," Chapter 2 discusses breast cancer in men. Readers will receive a thorough introduction to the illness in this chapter, which will cover the several varieties of breast cancer that can affect men, risk factors that raise a man's risk of getting the disease, and its causes.

The chapter will also review the warning signs and symptoms of breast cancer in males, such as lumps or swelling in the breast tissue, nipple changes, and skin changes around the breast. The significance of being aware of changes in one's breast tissue and acting quickly if they see anything unexpected will be stressed to readers.

In addition to reviewing the fundamentals of breast cancer in males, this chapter will also examine the numerous risk factors. Among them include possible genetic alterations, radiation exposure, liver disease, and a family history of breast cancer. Readers will learn how crucial it is to be aware of their unique risk factors and take action to lower their risk of acquiring breast cancer.

In the chapter's final section, we'll discuss the various breast cancers that might affect males, such as invasive ductal carcinoma and invasive lobular carcinoma. The author will discuss the characteristics of each type of breast cancer, as well as their detection and management. At the end of the chapter, readers will thoroughly understand the fundamentals of breast cancer in males and how to recognize and diagnose the condition.

Types Of Male Breast Cancer

Various forms of breast cancer affect men, including:

A non-invasive form of breast cancer called ductal carcinoma in situ (DCIS) begins in the breast's milk ducts. Male breast cancer is most frequently DCIS.

Breast cancer of the invasive ductal carcinoma (IDC) variety begins in the breast's milk ducts and invades the surrounding tissue. Invasive breast cancer in men is most frequently IDC.

A kind of breast cancer called invasive lobular carcinoma (ILC) develops in the lobules, the breast's milk-producing glands. In males, ILC is less frequent than IDC.

A rare form of breast cancer called Paget's disease of the nipple begins in the breast's ducts and spreads to the skin around the areola and nipple.

Inflammatory breast cancer: This rare and aggressive form of breast cancer can affect men. It causes the breast to swell, turn red, and feel warm.

The prognosis and course of treatment for each form of breast cancer might differ. It is crucial to remember this. Men with breast cancer should consult carefully with their medical team to choose the most effective treatment.

Danger Signs

Males are more likely to get breast cancer due to several risk factors. They comprise:

Age: Men over 60 accounts for most breast cancer cases in males, who are more likely to develop it as they age.

Family history: Males are more likely to contract the disease if there is a history of breast cancer in a first-degree relative (parent, sibling, or kid).

Mutations in particular genes, such as BRCA1 and BRCA2, can raise a man's risk of breast cancer.

Radiation exposure: There may be an increased risk of breast cancer in men exposed to radiation, especially in the chest region.

Hormone imbalances: Males who suffer from illnesses that alter their hormone levels, such as Klinefelter syndrome or liver cirrhosis, may be more likely to develop breast cancer.

Alcohol consumption: Drinking too much alcohol can increase a man's risk of breast cancer.

Overweight or obese men may be at higher risk of acquiring breast cancer.

It's crucial to remember that a man is not getting breast cancer just because he has one or more risk factors. The signs and symptoms of breast cancer should be known to men, and they should also undergo routine screening and monitoring by a medical expert if they have one or more risk factors.

Causes Of Male Breast Cancer

There is still much to learn about the precise causes of breast cancer in men. Research, however, indicates that breast cancer in men may frequently result from alterations (mutations) in the DNA of breast cells. These mutations may result in uncontrollable cell growth and division, which might result in the growth of a tumor.

A man's risk of breast cancer may increase because of risk factors that enhance the likelihood of DNA mutations, including aging, family history, and radiation exposure. But a lot of male breast cancer instances happen without any identified risk factors.

It's crucial to understand that contrary to popular belief, males do not develop breast cancer through using deodorants, wearing tight clothing, or any other widespread fallacies. Obesity and alcohol consumption are two lifestyle choices that may raise the risk of getting breast cancer, although they are not the actual causes of the condition.

symptoms and indications

Male breast cancer symptoms and indicators can include:

A bulge or enlargement in the breast, frequently close to the nipple

Clear, red, or another hue may be present in the nipple discharge.

Negative nipple (when the nipple turns inward)

Breast skin that has dimples or wrinkles

The skin on the breast or nipple may exhibit redness or scaling.

In the armpit, swollen lymph nodes

Breast discomfort or sensitivity is crucial to keep in mind that these signs and symptoms could also be brought on by other illnesses, such as a breast infection or benign (non-cancerous) breast growth. However, any alterations to the breast or nipple should be examined by a medical expert to ascertain the underlying cause.

Because it is uncommon, male breast cancer frequently goes undetected until it has advanced to a more advanced stage. To guarantee early detection and treatment of any potential breast cancer, men who observe any changes in their nipples or breast should contact a doctor right once.

Chapter 3

Diagnosis and Staging

Men are often diagnosed with breast cancer using a combination of physical examinations, imaging studies, and biopsies. Staging is done to evaluate the degree of cancer and help inform treatment choices after breast cancer has been detected.

The following subjects will be covered in this chapter:

Physical examinations: These examinations could involve a lymph node exam, a clinical breast exam, and a breast exam.

Imaging tests: Imaging procedures, including mammography, ultrasound, and MRI, can be used to find breast cancer and pinpoint the size and location of the tumor.

Breast tissue is removed for a biopsy, which entails analyzing it under a microscope to check for the presence of cancer cells.

Staging: Staging is the process of figuring out how far cancer has traveled throughout the body and how much it has grown. The size of the tumor, the quantity of affected lymph nodes, and the presence of distant metastases are some of the parameters that determine the staging.

To aid in guiding treatment choices and ascertain the likelihood of cancer recurrence, additional tests, such as genetic testing, may be advised.

Men with breast cancer can collaborate closely with their healthcare team to create a personalized treatment plan that takes into account the particulars of their cancer by being aware of the diagnostic and staging procedures.

Male breast cancer screening

Since that men are significantly less likely than women to develop breast cancer, normal healthcare does not typically include screening for the disease. Nonetheless, regular breast cancer screening may be beneficial for men who are at higher risk of getting breast cancer due to family history, genetic abnormalities, or other causes.

Male breast cancer screening may include the following:

Men can conduct routine breast self-examinations to look for any changes in the breast or nipple.

Clinical breast exams: To look for lumps or other abnormalities in the breast, a healthcare professional might conduct a clinical breast exam as part of a standard physical examination.

Mammography: A breast check using X-rays, mammography can identify breast cancer in both men and women. Yet, because men's breast tissue differs from women's in terms of density and structure, mammography is less effective in males than in women.

Additional imaging tests: Mammography may be combined with other imaging procedures, such as ultrasound or MRI, to help diagnose breast cancer in males.

Men who are more likely to get breast cancer may benefit from talking to their doctor about breast cancer screening. Depending on a person's risk factors and medical history, different screening tests may be advised at different intervals and for different purposes.

Diagnostic Procedures

Physical examinations, imaging exams, and biopsies may be used as diagnostic procedures for male breast cancer. These tests are used to identify and classify breast cancer as well as gauge its severity.

Physical examinations: A healthcare provider may do a physical examination of the breast to look for any tumors or anomalies in the breast or nipple.

Clinical breast exam: During a clinical breast exam, a medical expert looks for lumps or other abnormalities in the breast tissue and the lymph nodes that surround it.

Imaging tests: Imaging procedures including mammography, ultrasound, and MRI can be used to find breast cancer and pinpoint the size and location of the tumor.

Breast tissue is removed for a biopsy, which entails analyzing it under a microscope to check for the presence of cancer cells. There are various kinds of biopsies, such as:

A sample of cells from the breast is taken using a fine-needle aspiration biopsy.

A bigger needle is used for a core needle biopsy, which involves taking a small sample of tissue from the breast.

Surgical biopsy: To remove a larger portion of tissue from the breast, surgery is required.

To assist in guiding treatment choices and figuring out the likelihood of cancer recurrence, other tests, such as genetic testing, may be advised.

The process of diagnosing breast cancer often includes diagnostic tests, which help evaluate the presence and stage of the disease as well as inform treatment choices. To ensure early detection and treatment of any potential breast cancer, men should seek medical assistance as soon as they observe any changes in their nipple or breast.

Breast Cancer Grading And Staging

The diagnosis and management of breast cancer in men involve staging and grading. While grading relates to the look and behavior of the cancer cells, staging refers to the size and spread of the tumor.

Staging:

The TNM staging approach, which stands for tumor, node, and metastasis, is generally used for breast cancer staging in men. This procedure considers the tumor's size, if the malignancy has migrated to neighboring lymph nodes, and whether it has affected other bodily regions.

For men, the stages of breast cancer are:

Stage 0: The breast has abnormal cells, but they haven't migrated to the lymph nodes or adjacent tissue.

Stage I: The tumor is small and has not metastasized to the lymph nodes close by.

Stage II: A bigger tumor or lymph nodes nearby have been affected.

Stage III: A sizable tumor that has migrated to adjacent lymph nodes or other tissues, like the skin or chest wall.

Stage IV: The cancer has progressed to the bones, liver, or lungs, among other organs.

Grading:

The Nottingham histologic grading method, which considers the appearance of the cancer cells under a microscope, is frequently used to grade breast cancer in men. Depending on the level of abnormalities of the cancer cells, the grading method offers a score between 1 and 3.

The results are:

Grade 1: The cancer cells have the closest resemblance to healthy breast cells and are less likely to quickly multiply and spread.

Grade 2: The cancer cells have a somewhat aberrant appearance and may develop and proliferate more quickly.

Grade 3: The cancer cells have a very aberrant appearance and have a higher propensity to proliferate quickly.

While choosing the right course of treatment for males with breast cancer, staging and grading are crucial considerations. When creating a treatment plan, the healthcare team will consider the patient's overall health and preferences in addition to the stage and grade of the cancer.

Chapter 4

Alternatives for therapy

Typically, surgery, radiation treatment, chemotherapy, and hormone therapy are used to treat breast cancer in men. The particular course of treatment will be determined by the cancer's grade and stage, as well as the patient's general health and preferences.

Surgery: When a man has breast cancer, surgery is frequently his initial course of action. Surgery aims to eliminate the tumor and any surrounding tissue. A partial mastectomy, sometimes known as a lumpectomy, or a mastectomy (removal of the entire breast), depending on the severity of the cancer, may be advised.

High-energy rays are used in radiation therapy to eliminate cancer cells. After surgery, it may be used to eliminate any cancer cells that remain and lower the likelihood of a recurrence.

Chemotherapy: Drugs are used in chemotherapy to eradicate cancer cells throughout the body. It can be used either before or after surgery to shrink the tumor or eradicate any cancer cells that may still be present.

Hormone therapy: Hormone therapy is used to prevent the release or effect of hormones like estrogen, which can promote the growth of some kinds of breast cancer. It can be applied either alone or in conjunction with other therapies to treat hormone receptor-positive breast cancer.

Targeted therapy: A type of treatment that specifically targets chemicals or pathways that support the growth and division of cancer cells. For some kinds of breast cancer, it can be used either alone or in conjunction with other therapies.

Men with breast cancer may also gain from supportive care, which includes counseling, dietary support, and pain management, in addition to these treatments. Working closely with their medical team, men with breast cancer should create a specialized treatment plan that takes into account their unique requirements and preferences.

Surgery

Male breast cancer patients frequently have surgery. Surgery aims to remove the malignant tumor as well as any potentially cancerous tissue from its surroundings. The size and stage of the tumor, as well as the patient's general condition, will determine the kind of surgery that is advised.

Men with breast cancer can undergo one of two primary surgical procedures:

In a lumpectomy, commonly referred to as a partial mastectomy, the cancerous tumor plus a small portion of the surrounding tissue are removed. In cases of early-stage breast cancer in men where the tumor is tiny and has not yet spread to adjacent lymph nodes, this is usually advised.

Mastectomy: During a mastectomy, the entire breast is removed. Larger tumors, those located in hard-to-treat regions, or tumors where cancer has spread to adjacent lymph nodes are often advised for this.

When determining whether cancer has spread to the lymph nodes, a sentinel lymph node biopsy may be carried out during surgery in some instances. In order to do this, a select few lymph nodes that get drainage from the tumor location initially must be removed.

Men with breast cancer who have undergone surgery can also require radiation therapy, chemotherapy, hormone therapy, or targeted therapy in the future. Working closely with the medical team will help you choose the best course of action and manage any potential side effects from surgery or other treatments.

Radiation Treatment

High-energy radiation is used in radiation therapy to eliminate cancer cells. After surgery, it is frequently used to eliminate any cancer cells that may still be present and lower the likelihood of a recurrence. To treat males with more advanced forms of breast cancer, radiation therapy may also be combined with additional therapies including chemotherapy or hormone therapy.

A machine administers high-energy radiation to the breast's afflicted area during radiation therapy. Typically, the treatment is administered daily over the course of a few weeks. Fatigue, skin irritability, and breast soreness or swelling are possible side effects of radiation therapy.

In general, radiation therapy for breast cancer in men is both effective and safe. But, it's crucial to go over the advantages and hazards with a healthcare professional. If the hazards outweigh the benefits, radiation therapy may not be advised in specific situations, such as in older men or those with underlying medical issues.

Chemotherapy

Chemotherapy is a medical procedure that employs chemicals to eradicate cancer cells all over the body. It can be used either before or after surgery to shrink the tumor or eradicate any cancer cells that may still be present. For males with more advanced forms of breast cancer, chemotherapy may also be combined with additional therapies like radiation therapy or hormone therapy.

Chemotherapy medications are frequently administered in cycles with breaks in between to give the body time to heal. The medications can be taken orally or intravenously (via an IV). The kind and stage of the patient's breast cancer, as well as their general health, will determine the precise medications utilized and the length of the treatment.

Chemotherapy's side effects might include diarrhea, vomiting, hair loss, exhaustion, and a higher risk of infection. Chemotherapy can destroy cancer cells, but it also has the potential to harm healthy cells, which can have negative repercussions. Supportive care, such as painkillers or nausea medications, can lessen these adverse effects, nevertheless.

Working closely with a medical team will help you choose the best chemotherapy plan and manage any potential adverse effects. In rare circumstances, if chemotherapy is not suitable or effective, alternate treatments could be suggested.

Hormone Treatment

A treatment called hormone therapy counteracts the effects of hormones like estrogen and testosterone that may promote the growth of breast cancer cells. It is primarily utilized in male breast cancer patients who have cancer cells that have estrogen or progesterone receptors.

There are numerous ways to provide hormone treatment, including through medicine or surgery. Selective estrogen receptor modulators (SERMs), aromatase inhibitors, and luteinizing hormone-releasing hormone (LHRH) agonists are some of the drugs utilized in hormone treatment. These drugs can either lessen the amount of estrogen in the body or stop it from having an impact on cancerous cells.

The testicles, which are a major source of testosterone in men, may occasionally be surgically removed. It's called an orchiectomy.

Hot flashes, exhaustion, a decline in sex drive, and mood swings are some side effects of hormone therapy. Hormone therapy can, however, be useful in lowering the chance of cancer recurrence and is typically well tolerated.

It is crucial to go over the advantages and disadvantages of hormone therapy with a healthcare professional, as well as any possible interactions with other prescription drugs or health issues.

Targeted Treatment

A type of cancer treatment called targeted therapy goes after particular chemicals that are involved in the development and spread of cancer cells. Targeted therapy minimizes harm to healthy cells by attempting to block or disrupt specific chemicals that are only present in cancer cells, as opposed to chemotherapy, which kills both healthy and diseased cells.

Men with breast cancer who have HER2/neu-positive cancer cells, which encourage the proliferation of cancer cells, may benefit from targeted therapy. Drugs used in targeted therapy that block the HER2 protein, such as trastuzumab and epratuzumab, can reduce or stop the proliferation of cancer cells.

The common delivery methods for targeted therapy are intravenously or orally, with a range of treatment times. The potential side effects of targeted therapy include infection risk, tiredness, nausea, and diarrhea.

Working closely with a medical team will help you choose the most focused therapy plan and manage any side effects that could occur. To increase the effectiveness of the treatment, targeted therapy may occasionally be combined with additional therapies like radiation therapy or chemotherapy.

Chapter 5

Handling Therapy Adverse Effects

While cancer treatments can be successful in curing male breast cancer, they also carry a number of risks. Typical therapeutic side effects could include:

nausea and diarrhea

Fatigue

hair fall

reduced appetite

Skin sensitivity

oral sores

higher chance of infection

Sexually inappropriate

Lymphedema (swelling in the arms or legs) (swelling in the arms or legs)

Controlling these side effects is a crucial step in the healing process. Here are some guidelines for dealing with typical side effects:

Medicines can aid with nausea and vomiting management. Little, frequent meals and avoiding pungent odors may also be beneficial.

Fatigue: To assist manage weariness, take a break when necessary and attempt to exercise frequently.

Hair loss: Think about covering your head with a hat, scarf, or wig. Avoid using harsh hair products or shampoos.

Use gentle soaps and lotions on your skin, and stay out of the sun.

Mouth sores: Avoid foods that are hot or spicy, and maintain good oral hygiene.

Increased risk of infection: Avoid contact with sick people and wash your hands frequently.

Discuss treatment alternatives with a healthcare professional for sexual dysfunction.

Exercise, massage therapy, and the use of compression sleeves can all assist control of lymphedema.

Any side effects that occur while receiving treatment should be discussed with a healthcare professional. They may be able to modify treatment plans to lessen side effects and offer advice on how to manage problems.

Treatment-Related Physical Side Effects Of Breast Cancer

Depending on the type and length of treatment, breast cancer treatment may have a variety of physical adverse effects. Some typical physical adverse effects of breast cancer treatment are listed below:

Fatigue is a common side effect of breast cancer treatment and may be brought on by a number of different things, including chemotherapy, radiation therapy, surgery, and hormone therapy.

Hair loss: Chemotherapy may result in hair loss on the scalp, brows, and other body areas.

Lymphedema: Swelling in the arms, legs, or other regions of the body can result after surgery or radiation therapy to the lymph nodes, which can lead to a buildup of lymphatic fluid.

Chemotherapy and several other treatments can make you nauseous and make you want to throw up.

Skin changes: Radiation therapy can lead to skin changes in the treated area, such as redness, irritation, and dryness.

Infertility: Some medical procedures, such as chemotherapy or hormone therapy, might result in either temporary or permanent infertility.

Pain: Pain and discomfort are common side effects of surgery, radiation treatment, and chemotherapy that can be controlled with drugs and other treatments.

It is crucial to inform a medical staff of any physical adverse effects that occur while receiving treatment. They may be able to modify treatment plans to lessen side effects and offer advice on how to manage problems.

Psychological And Emotional Effects

Men may experience emotional and psychological side effects from breast cancer treatment. They may consist of:

Men with breast cancer frequently develop anxiety and sadness, which can be brought on by the diagnosis itself, the course of therapy, and future apprehension.

difficulties with body image: Men may experience self-consciousness over physical changes to their appearance, such as hair loss or surgical scarring.

Sexual dysfunction: A man's libido and sexual function may be impacted by procedures like surgery or hormone therapy.

Fear of recurrence: Men may be concerned that the cancer will come back or spread to another area of their bodies.

Financial worries: Cancer treatment can be costly and lead to stress over money.

Men may experience social isolation as a result of the stigma associated with male breast cancer.

Male breast cancer patients must put their emotional and psychological health first. To do this, for example:

asking friends, family, or a support group for help.

speaking with a therapist or mental health expert.

practicing stress-reduction techniques like meditation or exercise.

putting feelings into words or creating art.

To feel more in control, educate oneself on the illness and available treatments.

Have a conversation with a financial counselor to handle charges and worries.

In order to retain a high quality of life, it is crucial to be aware of the emotional and psychological side effects of breast cancer therapy.

Coping mechanisms and available resources

Managing the emotional and psychological effects of the disease can be difficult for men with breast cancer, but there are numerous services available to assist. Consider the following coping techniques and sources of support:

Speak to family and friends and ask for their support. Speak to family and friends and ask for their support. Stress can be reduced by communicating your feelings honestly and openly.

Join a support group: Meeting people who are going through the same thing might be found in support groups. Groups, whether online or in person, can offer information, guidance, and emotional support.

A mental health professional or therapist can assist you in developing coping mechanisms to manage the emotional and psychological effects of breast cancer. Take into consideration counseling or therapy.

Self-care is important. Make sure to look after your physical and emotional needs. This includes obtaining enough rest, following a healthy diet, and taking part in enjoyable activities.

Learn as much as you can about breast cancer and the available treatments so that you can feel more in control of your situation.

Seek financial assistance: Because breast cancer treatment can be costly, it's vital to look into any financial aid that may be available. The following are some resources for males with breast cancer:

The Male Breast Cancer Coalition is a group that supports, informs, and advocates on behalf of males with breast cancer.

Cancer Care is a national nonprofit organization that offers those impacted by cancer free counseling, support groups, information, and financial support.

For males with breast cancer, the American Cancer Society offers a wealth of resources, including details on diagnosis, care, and support options.

For males with breast cancer, the National Breast Cancer Foundation provides a hotline, patient guidance, and financial aid programs.

Always keep in mind that overcoming breast cancer is a journey, and it's crucial to discover what works best for you. Don't be afraid to ask for assistance and resources along the journey.

Chapter 6

Breast Cancer Afterlife

Men may experience difficulties adjusting to life following breast cancer treatment as they go through the disease. This chapter will go through some of the problems that males could run into as well as management techniques.

After treatment, it's crucial to keep up with routine check-ups with your doctor to keep an eye out for any signs of recurrence.

Physical recovery: Breast cancer therapy can be physically taxing, so it might take some time to go back to normal. When you restore strength, it's critical to pay attention to your body and pace yourself.

Emotional recovery: Many men with breast cancer continue to have emotional and psychological repercussions even after treatment. Emotional rehabilitation can be aided by looking for support from a therapist, support group, or loved ones.

Handling long-term side effects: Some men may develop persistent pain or lymphedema as a result of their treatment for breast cancer. These adverse effects can be managed with the assistance of a physical therapist and healthcare professional.

Body image and intimacy: A man's body image and sexual function may be impacted by physical changes to his body, such as scarring or hair loss. Discussing coping mechanisms for these changes with a counselor or medical professional could be beneficial.

Fear of recurrence: Cancer survivors frequently worry about their disease returning. Self-care activities and coping mechanisms can be used to control anxiety and terror.

Lifestyle modifications: Adopting a healthy lifestyle can assist to improve general health and lower the chance of cancer recurrence. Examples of such changes include frequent exercise and a balanced diet.

Awareness-raising efforts and advocacy for research and services for male breast cancer are made by many men who are diagnosed with the disease.

Life after breast cancer can often be a time of growth and adjustment. Men who receive therapy can lead happy lives with the correct assistance and tools.

Supplied care

Men often continue to see their doctor for routine follow-up care even after their breast cancer treatment is over. Depending on a person's unique circumstances, the frequency and kind of follow-up care may vary, however the following are some common objectives:

identifying and treating any new or recurring breast cancer

managing any treatment's lingering negative effects

keeping an eye out for any treatment-related long-term side effects, like heart or lung issues

providing resources and emotional support

At follow-up visits, the medical professional may do physical examinations, request blood tests or imaging studies, and talk with the patient about any symptoms or worries they may have. Men should inform their doctor of any new or unusual symptoms, such as changes in breast tissue, lumps or bumps, pain, or other signs and symptoms.

Men should continue to practice healthy lifestyle choices, such as exercise and a balanced diet, in addition to routine follow-up checkups, to maintain general health and lower the risk of cancer recurrence. Also, they must be informed about the recommended cancer screening procedures for various cancers, including prostate or colon cancer.

Lastly, to address any emotional or psychological concerns linked to their breast cancer diagnosis and treatment, men may find it helpful to join a support group or seek counseling. A healthcare professional can offer resources for assistance and counseling.

Restoration and retraining

Men who have undergone treatment for breast cancer should prioritize their recovery and rehabilitation. Men may undergo physical, mental, and psychological changes that may have an impact on their general quality of life as a result of breast cancer treatment, which can be physically taxing on the body.

The following are some methods for healing and rehabilitation:

Relaxation and recuperation: After treatment, it's crucial to give your body time to rest and heal. To do this, you might reduce your workload or take time off from work, in addition to obtaining enough rest and taking breaks as necessary.

Exercise: Regular exercise can enhance mood, reduce fatigue, and improve physical function. Start with low-impact exercises like walking or swimming and discuss safe exercise regimens with your healthcare provider.

Nutrition: Consuming a balanced, healthy diet helps promote general well-being and lower the chance of cancer recurrence. Put an emphasis on complete foods, such as fresh produce, whole grains, and lean protein.

Management of lymphedema: Lymphedema is a frequent side effect of breast cancer treatment that can result in arm or chest swelling. Exercises and management methods might be given by a physical therapist to aid with lymphedema.

Body image and sexual function may be impacted by physical changes to the body, such as scarring or hair loss. You might find it easier to deal with these changes if you talk to a therapist or counselor.

Emotional and mental well-being: After breast cancer therapy, many men may experience emotional and psychological repercussions. Emotional rehabilitation can be aided by looking for support from a therapist, support group, or loved ones.

It's crucial to keep in mind that each person's process of recovery and rehabilitation is different, and there is no universal strategy. You can create a tailored recovery plan that takes into account your unique requirements and goals by working with a healthcare professional, physical therapist, and other support providers.

Preventing A Repeat

The main objective of follow-up care for men who have finished their treatment for breast cancer is to prevent its recurrence. While there is no surefire strategy to stop cancer from returning, men can employ a number of strategies to lower their chance of recurrence.

Here are several methods for avoiding a recurrence of breast cancer:

Care after treatment: Keeping an eye out for any indications of cancer recurrence or the development of new cancers requires scheduling regular follow-up sessions with a healthcare professional. Attend all scheduled follow-up appointments, and notify your doctor of any new or unusual symptoms.

Changes in lifestyle: Choosing a healthy way of life can help lower the risk of cancer recurrence. This entails getting regular exercise, following a healthy diet, keeping a healthy weight, abstaining from tobacco use, and drinking too much alcohol.

Medication: Some men may benefit from taking medicine to lower their chance of developing cancer again. Depending on the individual's particular circumstances,

this can involve hormone therapy, chemotherapy, or targeted therapy.

Genetic testing: Some males may have a mutation in their genes that makes them more likely to get breast cancer. See your healthcare practitioner about genetic testing if you were diagnosed with breast cancer at an early age, have a family history of the disease, or have any other linked cancers.

Support from loved ones, attending support groups, or getting counseling can all assist to enhance mental well-being and lower the risk of a cancer recurrence. Emotional and psychological support.

Keep in mind that preventing cancer recurrence is a lifelong endeavor, therefore it's crucial to maintain contact with your doctor and lead a healthy lifestyle. You can lower your chance of cancer recurrence and enhance your general quality of life by taking an active part in your health and wellbeing.

Changes In Lifestyle For Long-Term Health

Living after breast cancer involves changing one's lifestyle for long-term health. Healthy lifestyle choices can enhance general health and wellbeing in addition to lowering the chance of cancer recurrence. Men can adopt the following lifestyle modifications to support long-term health:

Exercise frequently: Frequent exercise has several health advantages, including lowering the risk of chronic conditions like diabetes and heart disease. Try to exercise for at least 30 minutes, most days of the week, at a moderate level.

Have a balanced diet that is high in fruits, vegetables, whole grains, and lean proteins to help lower your chance of developing chronic diseases and improve your general health.

Keep a healthy weight: Obesity and overweight are linked to an increased risk of cancer and other chronic diseases. Long-term health depends on maintaining a healthy weight through nutrition and activity.

Reduce your alcohol intake because it raises your risk of developing various malignancies, including breast cancer. Men should limit their alcohol intake to two drinks per day at most.

Avoid tobacco usage: Smoking and other tobacco use are associated with a number of cancer types as well as other

chronic disorders. One of the best things a man can do for his long-term health is to stop smoking.

Control your stress: Prolonged stress can have detrimental impacts on your health, including raising your risk of developing chronic conditions like depression and heart disease. Long-term health can be improved by finding appropriate strategies to cope with stress, such as through exercise, meditation, or counseling.

Men can lower their chance of developing chronic diseases and improve their general health and well-being by adopting these healthy lifestyle choices. It's crucial to keep in mind that although making these changes requires time and work, they are worthwhile. Men can successfully navigate life after breast cancer and enjoy long-term health with the help of medical professionals, loved ones, and friends.

Chapter 7

Special Difficulties for Male Breast Cancer Patients

Male breast cancer patients could experience particular difficulties with the illness and its therapies. These difficulties may include:

Lack of knowledge and understanding: Because male breast cancer is relatively uncommon, there may be a lack of knowledge and understanding among the general public, medical professionals, and even male patients. This may make it more challenging to receive a prompt diagnosis and the best course of treatment.

Stigma and gender norms: Men who develop breast cancer may experience stigma and a sense of emasculation because it is frequently believed to be an illness that only affects women. Also, men may experience pressure to adhere to conventional gender roles, which can make it challenging for them to discuss breast cancer and seek help.

Concerns about sexual function and body image: Breast cancer and its treatment can have physical and mental repercussions that affect these two areas. Men may experience anxiety or sadness as a result of physical changes to their body, such as breast reduction surgery or weight increase.

Absence of support groups: Although there are support groups for breast cancer survivors, these organizations frequently target female members. Attending these meetings could make men uncomfortable, or they might not be able to locate a group that is particularly for men with breast cancer.

Work and financial worries: Breast cancer treatment may affect a man's capacity for work, which may cause stress and financial worries.

It's critical for men with breast cancer to address these issues and get the help they need. Healthcare professionals can offer men resources and information to assist them deal with the disease's and its treatment's physical and emotional repercussions. Addressing these issues and establishing connections with people who have gone through comparable situations can also be facilitated via counseling and support groups.

Managing The Stigma Associated With Male Breast Cancer

Although overcoming the stigma associated with breast cancer in men might be difficult, there are certain techniques that can be helpful:

Get knowledgeable about breast cancer in males, both for yourself and others. By doing so, you can lessen the stigma associated with the disease. To help others understand that breast cancer can afflict anyone, regardless of gender, you can also share your personal stories and experiences.

Establish a connection with others: Joining a support group or getting in touch with other men who have battled breast cancer can give you a sense of belonging and comprehension. Connecting with others can also be facilitated by participating in online forums and support groups.

Maintaining good physical and mental health will help you feel more in control and capable of handling the challenges brought on by breast cancer. This can involve maintaining a balanced diet, exercising frequently, and engaging in stress-relieving activities like yoga or meditation.

Get professional assistance: Seeing a therapist or counselor can offer a secure setting to explore your feelings around the stigma associated with breast cancer in males and to create coping mechanisms. Your healthcare physician may also be able to refer you to sources of information and support groups.

Advocate for change: Raising awareness of the stigma associated with breast cancer in males and pushing for more information and support can help lessen that stigma and enhance care for all people who are touched by breast cancer.

preserving one's self-worth and masculinity

Men with breast cancer may have serious concerns about maintaining their sense of manhood and self-worth. Here are some tactics that could be useful:

Read everything you can about breast cancer in males and realize that anyone can develop it, regardless of gender. You may feel more in control and capable of managing your diagnosis if you have a better understanding of the illness.

Pay attention to your assets: Remind yourself of your qualities and achievements that are independent of your diagnosis. Take part in activities you find enjoyable and that boost your self-esteem.

Look for support: Reaching out to other men who have experienced breast cancer or joining a support group can help you feel more connected and understanding. Discussing any emotions of guilt or loss of masculinity with a therapist or counselor can also be beneficial.

Talk to your spouse if you have one: If you do, it can be beneficial to talk openly and honestly to your partner about your worries and emotions. Education about male breast cancer may be beneficial for your partner as well.

Make sure you are getting adequate and considerate treatment from your healthcare professionals by acting as your own advocate. It's crucial to speak up and defend yourself if you feel uncomfortable or insulted.

Keep in mind that breast cancer does not determine your worth as a man or your manhood. While you navigate your diagnosis and treatment, it's crucial to concentrate on your strengths and get help.

Establishing A Support System

Developing a support system is important for males with breast cancer. Here are a few techniques to do it:

Involve your family and friends: Inform your loved ones about your condition and how they can support you. Ask for specifics like meals or rides to appointments.

Join a support group: Both general cancer support groups and organizations just for men with breast cancer are plentiful. This may present a chance to interact with people who can relate to what you're going through.

Get expert assistance: Think about visiting a therapist or counselor with knowledge of working with cancer patients. They can offer you emotional support, assist you in managing stress, and equip you with the means to deal with depression or anxiety.

Connect with online resources: Men with breast cancer can find a variety of online forums and resources. This can be a terrific method to obtain support and information while also connecting with people who are going through similar things.

Think about volunteering: A significant method to make friends and discover a feeling of purpose is by lending a hand to those who are experiencing similar things. Search for volunteer opportunities with cancer-related groups or at cancer treatment facilities.

Creating a support system takes time and effort, but it may be a crucial source of both emotional and practical help as you battle illness. Never be reluctant to ask for assistance when you need it.

Chapter 8

The Treatment of Breast Cancer in the Future

We will examine the most recent findings and innovations in the treatment of breast cancer in this chapter, including:

Immunotherapy: An approach to treating cancer that makes use of the immune system of the patient to combat the disease. Early results from research into immunotherapy as a potential breast cancer treatment are encouraging.

Precision medicine is a tailored method of treating cancer that takes into consideration both a patient's particular genetic profile and the particular features of their illness. Precision medicine is becoming a more realistic option for breast cancer patients thanks to developments in genetic testing and data analysis.

Targeted therapies that target particular proteins or genes involved in the growth and spread of cancer cells are among the innovative medication therapies for breast cancer that researchers are continually developing.

New screening techniques: Breast cancer screening is becoming more accurate and trustworthy thanks to developments in imaging technology and genetic testing, which may result in earlier detection and improved outcomes.

Artificial intelligence (AI): AI is used to analyze vast volumes of data to find trends and forecast results in the treatment of breast cancer. It is possible that this technology will increase the precision of diagnosis and treatment planning.

The future of breast cancer treatment appears bright as researchers make further advancements in the field. Men with breast cancer should stay up-to-date on new research and collaborate closely with their medical professionals to choose the best course of action for their particular circumstance.

Advancements In The Study And Treatment Of Breast Cancer

Recent advances in breast cancer research have led to more effective and novel treatment choices. Following are some of the most significant developments in the study and treatment of breast cancer:

Targeted therapy: A type of treatment known as targeted therapy targets particular molecules or proteins that are involved in the development and spread of cancer cells. This strategy has resulted in the creation of novel medications that can target breast cancer cells with precision while causing the least amount of harm to healthy cells.

Immunotherapy: An approach to treating cancer that makes use of the immune system of the patient to combat the disease. Particularly when used in conjunction with other therapies, it has demonstrated promise in the treatment of breast cancer.

Genetic testing: Genetic testing enables medical professionals to examine a patient's cancer cells' DNA in order to spot any specific genetic alterations that might be causing the tumor to grow. With this knowledge, customized treatment regimens that concentrate on those particular mutations can be created.

Surgery has made great strides in recent years, enabling more precise and minimally invasive operations. Less pain and quicker recovery times for patients have resulted as a result of this.

Radiation therapy has also advanced thanks to innovative methods that deliver more precise radiation dosages while causing the least amount of harm to healthy tissue.

Supporting care: As a crucial component of breast cancer therapy, supportive care now includes services including dietary counseling, pain management, and psychological support that assist patients in coping with side effects and enhancing their quality of life.

Further improvements in the detection and treatment of breast cancer are likely to be made as research proceeds, improving patient outcomes.

On the horizon are new treatments

For the treatment of breast cancer, various novel medicines are currently being studied, including:

CAR T-cell therapy: CAR T-cell therapy is an immunotherapy in which the immune system of the patient is altered to recognize and combat cancer cells. Early investigations on breast cancer using this method have yielded encouraging results.

PARP inhibitors: A particular protein that aids cancer cells in repairing DNA damage is blocked by this form of targeted therapy. Patients with specific genetic alterations, such as BRCA mutations, have demonstrated these medications to be effective in treating their breast cancer.

Bispecific antibodies are a type of targeted therapy that have the capacity to bind to two distinct targets simultaneously, which can improve their capacity to kill cancer cells. In clinical studies, several bispecific antibodies are being investigated for the treatment of breast cancer.

Immunomodulatory medications: A family of medications known as immunomodulatory medications can help control the immune system's reaction to cancer. Clinical trials for the treatment of breast cancer are now being conducted on several of these medications.

Nanoparticle-based therapies: These therapies give medication to cancer cells directly using small particles. This strategy may help chemotherapy work more effectively while minimizing negative effects.

Further research is required to determine the safety and efficacy of these novel medicines because they are still in the early phases of development. They do, however, give promise for future advancements in the breast cancer patient treatment options.

Chapter 9

CONCLUSION

In conclusion, men and women alike can be impacted by the serious illness known as breast cancer. Men who are diagnosed with breast cancer should work closely with their healthcare providers to create a unique treatment plan because early detection and treatment are essential to improving outcomes.

This book has given a general overview of male breast cancer, covering risk factors, symptoms, diagnostic procedures, and available treatments. Additionally, it discussed coping mechanisms for the particular difficulties that men with breast cancer may experience.

Last but not least, we discussed some of the innovative new medicines being created for the treatment of breast cancer and emphasized the significance of continuous research in this field. We can aspire to enhance the prognosis and quality of life for men with breast cancer with ongoing research and treatment advancements.

Last thoughts and words of inspiration

Please know that you are not alone if you are a man who has been diagnosed with breast cancer. It's crucial to keep in mind that breast cancer does not define you and that, with the correct care and assistance, you can beat this condition.

Take responsibility for your health and collaborate closely with your medical team to create a treatment plan that is suited to your particular requirements. Keep up with new developments in research and treatment choices, and don't be shy about seeking clarification or more information.

Always remember to look after your physical and mental needs, and when necessary, seek out support from loved ones, friends, and support groups. You can beat breast cancer and lead a healthy, full life with willpower, bravery, and support.

Resources For Breast Cancer In Men

Male breast cancer patients have access to a number of resources. To name a few:

The Male Breast Cancer Coalition is a group that offers information, activism, and support to men who have breast cancer. They provide peer-to-peer support programs, support groups, and internet resources.

The American Cancer Society: This group offers information and resources, such as treatment alternatives, support services, and survivorship resources, for men with breast cancer.

Men with breast cancer can access a variety of tools from Life Beyond Breast Cancer, including webinars, support groups, and online discussion boards.

For persons with cancer and their loved ones, Cancer Care provides free counseling, support groups, and informational materials.

The National Cancer Institute is a source of information on breast cancer, including available therapies, scientific studies, and clinical trials.

For males with breast cancer, these resources can be a great source of knowledge, assistance, and community.

Crucial Words Glossary

The following are essential words in relation to breast cancer:.

- Chemotherapy: A medical procedure that employs chemicals to destroy cancer cells.
- Hormone therapy: A method of treating cancer that inhibits or eliminates hormones to decrease the proliferation of cancer cells.
- Surgery to simply remove the malignant tumor and some surrounding tissue is known as a lumpectomy.
- Mammogram: A breast X-ray used to look for breast cancer.

An entire breast is removed during a mastectomy.

Cancer metastasizing: When cancer spreads from one area of the body to another.

High-energy radiation is used in radiation therapy to eliminate cancer cells.

- Stage: The amount of a cancer's internal spread.

A tumor is an abnormal development of tissue that may or may not be cancerous (benign).

- prognosis describes the likely course or result of an illness.
- An oncologist is a medical professional who focuses on the treatment of cancer.
- An operation to remove the first lymph node(s) where cancer is most likely to spread from the main tumor is known as a sentinel lymph node biopsy.